D0856531

AMPUTATIONS

THE BRAZILLER SERIES OF POETRY
Richard Howard, General Editor

T.

AMPUTATIONS

Poems by

CYNTHIA MACDONALD

with a note by Richard Howard

GEORGE BRAZILLER

New York

Some of these poems have previously appeared in the following publications, to whose editors grateful acknowledgment is made: "Paintings from the Slaughterhouse: A Slide Show of Hogs" and "Instruction from Bly" have appeared in THE NEW AMERICAN REVIEW; "A Family Question" has appeared in THE NEW YORK QUARTERLY.

For information, address the publisher:
George Braziller, Inc.
One Park Avenue, New York 10016
Standard Book Number: 8076–0656–1, cloth
8076–0655–3, paper
Library of Congress Catalog Card Number: 72–80734
First Printing
Designed by Harry Ford and Kathleen Carey
Printed in the United States of America

With thanks and affection to:

Norman B. Hirt
Earle Birney

Alan Dugan
Jane Cooper

Barbara Greenwald
Janet Krauss

and especially Mac,
Timmie and Scott.

I wish to express my gratitude to Yaddo where some of these poems were written.

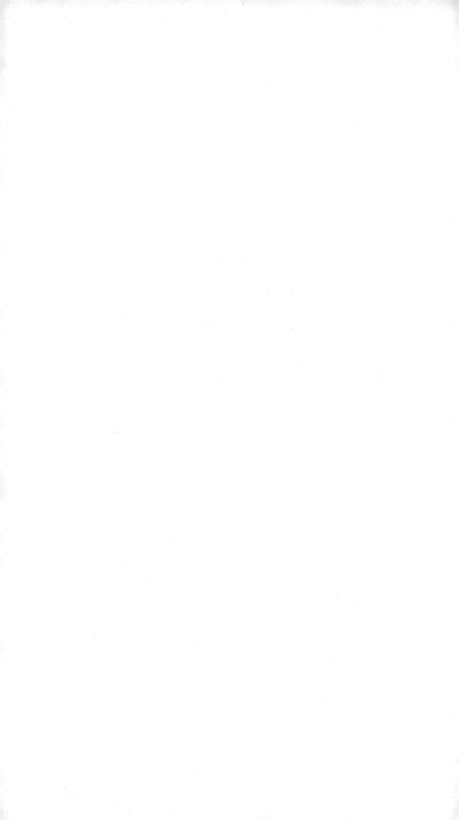

Contents

IV

CYNTHIA MACDONALD

. . . Years in which to become detached.

She had, like the rest of us, to start somewhere, and luckily for her poetry, Mrs. Macdonald started late. Of course there is no such thing as a late start or an early one in poetry, that is no more than a critical convenience, no less than a critical fiction, for there is no starting, there is only coming out, coming up, *reaching the surface* from somewhere which is not the surface—subcutaneous, ventral, deep; nor is there an end, poems are not finished but excused, and what matters is the terms between starting and finishing, or between the excursion and the excuse, the armistice between torment and terminal which is acceptable to both sides. So what I mean by a late start in Cynthia Macdonald's case is that she started *as* Mrs. Macdonald, as a mother twice over, as a woman who has been around, specifically, the world; and I mean that she got a *head* start, as well as a diaphragmal one, by becoming a musician, a singer, a professional performer. She learned, that is, the shape of a made thing not of her own making, yet which had to be produced or made over by her as if it *were* her own. She learned cunning, therefore, and she learned compliance—invaluable resources for a poet—and she learned, as it has turned out, how the appearance of the random must somewhere join the reality of contrivance. Then she started writing her poetry.

Of course it is musical, but in the formal sense in which poetry can be musical, not in the accidental and careless way in which we say that poetry is musical because it labors the sounds of vowels and by imposing a grid or pattern upon them keeps us from advancing *through* them. The poetry of *Amputations* is musical in the strict sense: it resolves a series or sequence of discords, it accounts for and enables movement, it moves onward, and its diction, as Northrop Frye says of all truly musical diction, is better fitted for the grotesque and horrible, or for invective and abuse. It is irregular in meter, leans heavily on enjambment, and employs a long cumulative rhythm sweeping the lines up into larger rhythmical units such as the paragraph.

It is poetry of a particular kind, then, and all of one kind—not uniform but unified, collected from experience which has sunk in. Or else it has originated wherever *in* may be. What is significant about this poetry is that it has moved from its origin or source (being, then, no longer merely original but resourceful), has reached what I have called the surface—nothing less than the eye, the ear, *other people*— and in performing this trajectory, it has had every occasion to discover its own nature, to *reveal itself*. What had been held down is now held up to utterance, the voice raised, brought from the un-sounded center to the circumference of expression, that part of our lives where things *take shape*.

Hence the ideogrammic or iconographic aspect of most of her poems, their design on the page being a design upon us: the page is the arena, the circus, the stage. The work of Cynthia Macdonald figures itself out, there, as the barker's pitch, leaves from the sibyl's cookbook, the diva's farewell—undertaken by necessity, overtaken by prowess— the vaudeville turn, earthworks, the *lazzo* of Commedia dell' Arte, and—I hope I have got the right sow by the ear—the commentary for a suburban chatauqua travelogue (splendors of Iowa); out of these unlikely *numbers*, which is after all the old name for poetry, she has made up her *sum*, which is after all the old name for a result reached by coming out on top, at the *summit* (the Romans counted upward), as well as a Latin word meaning what all poetry means: *I am*. The arithmetical processes employed here are the ones the Walrus used in the School of Fishes: *ambition, distraction, uglification* and *derision* —with some other additions to the curriculum in the form of *mystery, ancient and modern, drawling, stretching, and fainting in coils*, and of course the classical subjects *laughing* and *grief*. It amounts to saying that Cynthia Macdonald is a poet of the grotesque.

It is the wrong preposition. What I mean is that she is a poet *from* the grotesque. For by the grotesque we mean—the *language* means— something to do with the grotto, the originating cavern (womb, skull, lung) where it all starts. We call it the unconscious, that place where Lord knows what could be daubed on the walls of *living rock*, and where the goings-on, by smoky torchlight, were anything but edifying. The point is to get *out* of the grotto with that dark or dubious knowledge intact, to examine by some other illumination what could not be dealt with by the light of day. The unconscious is exciting, as we know from our dreams, but not interesting, as we know from other people's dreams. The conscious is interesting, as we know from other people's words, but it is not exciting, as we know from our own. What is both interesting and exciting is the passage from dreams to words, from the unconscious to the conscious. A poetry *of* the grotesque would be worthless, for we could not tell what we had; a poetry *from* the grotesque is what we have here, a cast of experience seized as it proceeds from the cave, out into sunlight.

Mrs. Macdonald's stratagem is generally to suppose that the worst has happened, to divine the consequences, as if the worst were not what does happen:

Today I rejoice: I even treat myself kindly
Because I have uncovered a crucial self-secret:
The reason for my defective memory, the why of my forgetting . . .

And then she proceeds, she gets on with it as if the worst were not to be shut back in the grotto, as it is by most of us, but were to be lived with, on and on, an ordinary evening in Purgatory. As she says, in another (awful) context, but with immense bearing on her poetry:

> I have more subjects than I can handle,
> But only volunteers. It is an art like hypnosis
> Which cannot be imposed on the unwilling victim.

She constitutes herself the willing victim, and her poems are reports—spiels, arias, inventories, laments, dirges, even eulogies—of the handling. There is an immense trajectory evident in her wit, in the delicacy of her phrasing, in the distinction of her ironies, in the sharpness of her ear for caste and class, for circumstantial "placing"—a vast parabola between what lies or lurks behind her and what she has made it into up front. By hilarious management, or one might say by a cool hand, she has taken the *terribilità* of her experience and made it, merely, operatic—which is to say that she has *worked* on it enough to make it ours, which is again to say that she has made it unmistakably, recognizably hers.

One word more. She has made it, also, prototypically American. There is nothing in her poetry which participates in the "international school"—half great plains, half grubby Paris—of easy surrealism being trumpeted (or kazooed) in some quarters. Mrs. Macdonald engages the capitalist realism of our culture from within, and her achievement can best be summarized or at least suggested by Hermann Broch's beautiful aphorism: "We are a *we*, not because we hold communion, but because our contours overlap."

RICHARD HOWARD

THE PLATFORM BUILDER

If you were to construct a platform,
    That is, if you wanted to construct a platform
  And then you did (after a lot of self-instruction
      On platform building and frequent consultation
  With the building supply people) and you worked
    Weekends till your friends, unobsessed with platforms,
    Stopped calling. And if, then, you finally got it built,
With what an invasion of accomplishment you'd view it . . . The tools
Not even put away, but left beside the scaffolding,
    You'd buy three things you'd been wanting and thinking about
                                  buying
  And sit with an old friend to watch "The Shoeshine Boy" on TV
If it was on.

The next day, looking at your platform,
    You'd see the gap between the second and third planks
      And how the miters showed how many
  Times you had made corrections. If you made
Another platform, you'd fix those things. And in the thinking of
                                  another
      The need is there or maybe the need
      Made you think of it.
So you begin again. Of course, it is more difficult,
  Demanding a platform cantilevered on the first,
    A kind of step above a base.
You build it, with the foreseen result: like owners who correct
In every house they build the faults of the last one; the flaws are not
The same, but there are flaws.

With each successive platform, the skill increases
  And the demands increase beyond the increase of the skills;
The choice of wood, fitting without nails or glue, the curve

3

To change direction at the sixteenth level
  When, emerging above the trees, it's evident
  The direction chosen affords a view
Of the oil storage tanks instead of the sea.
And then, a few levels higher, the question whether wood at all
  Or plexiglass (acrophobia?) or steel (too cold in winter?),
  Etc. And, on the twenty-second level, having to stop completely
    For Zoning Board appeals because you've gone
Beyond the allowed height for an AA zone.
    And interviews, and manufacturers who want you to build
    Another just the same, using their product.

Young builders, contemplating platforms,
    Examine what you've done and ask you how
You did those first ones and sometimes you say you can't remember,
        Which is true, and sometimes you try
To think just how and answer with how you did the latest ones
    Or even how you think you're going to do the next,
If you find time to do it.
    And they imagine you content with, not so much what you've
                                                        made—
    They've heard of creative dissatisfaction—
  But that it's been accepted; that you can get money and more
Than money for a speech on "How I Build Platforms" and only
        Will be asked to set another date
If you get drunk and don't show up.

If you want to build a platform, and ask for my advice,
        I'll give it, but remember
    I can't remember back to where you are . . .
  I think I would use wood to start,
  To get the platform's natural connection.

4

White ash is strong and tough and has escape built in its name.
      I think I cannot say it better than to say
If I were about to start to build a platform,
I think I'd start with ash.

OBJETS D'ART

When I was seventeen, a man in the Dakar Station
Men's Room (I couldn't read the signs) said to me:
You're a real ball cutter. I thought about that
For months and finally decided
He was right. Once I knew that was my thing,
Or whatever we would have said in those days,
I began to perfect my methods. Until then
I had never thought of trophies. Preservation
Was at first a problem: pickling worked
But was a lot of trouble. Freezing
Proved to be the answer. I had to buy
A second freezer just last year; the first
Was filled with rows and rows of
Pink and purple lumps encased in Saran wrap.

I have more subjects than I can handle,
But only volunteers. It is an art like hypnosis
Which cannot be imposed on the unwilling victim.
If you desire further information about the process and
The benefits, please drop in any night from nine to twelve.
My place is east of Third on Fifty-sixth.
You'll know it by the three gold ones over the door.

INVENTORY

I carry a suitcase everywhere with me—and I mean everywhere.
It weighs between nineteen and eighty pounds depending
What I put inside.

> A down-filled pillow, a gray Army
> blanket, a package of Droste bitter
> orange chocolate, my tape recorder
> with a tape of *Der Freischütz*, boots,
> sea-water from Vancouver Bay, next
> rooms opened by Nemerov, Lotte Lehmann's
> "Ich" and my Grandmother's trunk.

The case is useful, but doesn't justify it; I can't
Justify it. I can only say I need it
Even if

> A down-filled pillow, a gray Army
> blanket, typewriter and Corrasable
> Bond, a bowl of agates from Saudi
> Arabia, popcorn, *Buddenbrooks*, pieces
> of a red glass DANGER sign on which
> I'd cut my knee when I was five
> and disobeyed and walked on Milton Road,
> three fur hats and my Grandmother's trunk.

It interferes. And it does. For example, yesterday afternoon
I met Gunther. I did not know him well, but liked
What I knew.
He asked me if I wanted to see the Whitney Show; I said yes.
At first he didn't seem to notice the suitcase (though
I knew it
Must be what he remembered best about me). Then he did—

I guess when I began dragging. He offered
To check it
And when I said no, to carry it, but I couldn't let him.
At dinner it prevented me, as it always does when
I sit in
A booth, from getting close to the table and I dribbled Marinara
Sauce over it and down my front. I definitely blame
That case for
Making me look messy. When we got in bed it was the same old story:
Three of us. To spell it out: my case gets between me
And friends, especially
If they are not agile or are easily bruised. He tried, but got
So tired he fell asleep. I felt confined and decided to
Stretch out in the bathtub.
It was cozy there after I'd fixed it up with my down-filled
Pillow and gray Army blanket. I took out Beowulf and
Some cordial cherries
And my radio and relaxed, thinking, as I so often had,
How well-prepared I am to make the best of
A bad situation.

> A down-filled pillow, a gray Army
> blanket, a hate note to the editor
> of a certain magazine, my radio,
> an empty cordial cherry box, Beowulf,
> a tube of Gunther's cobalt blue,
> my left-handed father's left index
> finger and my Grandmother's trunk.

It's true; it is really true; that *is* the case.

CONSULTATION

I asked the person I ask for help for help
In finding someone to assist me in making
A new dictionary, one which will do more than define.
It will make words for those which are anemic:
Beautiful, lovely, dreadful. Or misleading:
Cry or weep. Or inadequate: copulate, fornicate,
Have intercourse, fuck, etc. . . . words that will
Transfuse blood, pulse through the heart and lungs
Until they disappear and simply are.

She listened carefully to what I said I needed,
Then answered, "I think I may know someone
Who could assist you in your work. He is
A Greek whose English is not good, but adequate.
And Greek could be of use. I definitely know
That he is slow and careful, although his frequent
Catatonic periods could interfere with progress.
But one could think of them as resting times." She looked
At her appointment book, "I can't explain exactly why I feel
He is the one; my intuition tells me so."

I bit my lip, "He seems the perfect choice."
She looked concerned, "He is the best one I can think of,
But let me check my files." From a box she pulled
A lizard, a recording of *Fedora*, a heart
Which she indentified as that of a goat, a prism and
Three Japanese grave statues. "You see," she gestured
At the objects, "I really think my first choice was the best."
She offered me her phone to call the Greek. I,
Having nowhere else to turn, dialed. He answered,
"Spiros Malepopolous." I explained. "Thalassa,
Thalassa," he replied. I stared at the wine-dark carpet,
Watching a child with flippers try to thread a needle.

9

PIRANESI'S PIRANDELLO

One is the prisoner, the other the jailer;
Both are inside the prison looking through opposite slits
At *Home, Sweet Home* cross-stitched in neon tubing
Above the guarded gate. They are waiting for lunch or break-
Fast. Meals are starchy but not maggoty;
The jailer gets extra meat and sweet raisins
In the oatmeal: reward, two, three, four.
The dog predicts he will get both their bones.

The prisoner builds fires in the cell-center
And, by request, reads the future in flame for
Other inmates who weasel-up rewards:
Goose lard from Strasbourg Pâté,
Muffs, Noah's Ark in a bottle,
And a cut-to-size rug of plastic grass.
The fire separates into jets of orange and blue:
"Cold blue will be your future and orange,
Hot as the skin of the sun will be yours." The angry
Jailer drowns the sun with a bucket of water,
"Prediction's childish games must be replaced
With ice-cold showers." He eats his nails.
The dog eyes the prisoner, anticipating bone.

The warden orders: "Inmates and guards, change
Places: Hup, two, three, four.
Unlock cells, go in, hand over
Keys and gun, extra meat, sweet raisins,
Change your stripes. Now, let's all join in
From our new positions, three-part, a capella:
        This old man, he played three,
        He played knick, knack with my knee . . ."

The prisoner has made a computer out of the bed-frame,
Twelve spoons, the counters from a game of checkers,
Hearing-aid batteries and wire. "Science
Has the answer; if we could find the question."
The machine rattles its parts, then hums
In response to, "What's a sure way out of here?"
Click, two, three, four: "Become the warden."
"Dismantle it," says the jailer, "we need the checkers,
And anyway, science cannot match reincarnation
As future's lock-picker. That flea may be Mahatma Gandhi."
The dog looks at the cages; dreams of rib;
Looks at the jailer, the prisoner again:
Certain both will make good bones.

The mother and father do not get along.
She is dressed in pink velvet; he
In a brown suit. The house is called a Dutch
Colonial. The living room has a secretary and
A carpet like moss. There are two medium-
Size children, both girls. Everyone
Has blue eyes and they are all blonde except
The father who has light brown hair. They bend
Quite well, though they are not jointed. I think
They are wired. Most of the time they fight. The sisters
About who interrupted who and which
Toy belongs to which of them. They try
To pull out each other's hair, but it
Is firmly rooted. Their room is yellow and white
And frilled with organdy the way I wish mine was.
They kick each other almost every time they
Are awake and would be lumped and bruised if
They were not composition. Maybe I will paint
Black and blues on one. Perhaps if they
Had friends they would not always fight. I have asked
For friends, but I will have to wait until
Next Christmas, unless my grandmother brings them when
She comes to visit. The dining room has a chandelier
As sparkling as an earring. There is a maid, but she
Is too big to play with them. She really
Cannot do anything but be a maid.
I cut a hole in a wash cloth and made her a dress,
But the white maid-hat is part of her composition hair;
So you could see she was still the maid.
She is always complaining about her varicose veins. The hall
Wallpaper is the color of sky. I am not
Exactly sure why the mother and father do not
Get along. They fight sometimes about who

Interrupted who or why someone
Invested too much in something or whether they
Will be too early or too late for the dinner
Party. But mostly they do not fight, but also
They do not get along. The bathroom has
A tub and basin and toilet and towels, but no
Water. She is very beautiful, especially
When she wears her diamond earrings. Her children
Come in when she is dressing to go out
And watch her put them on. She is really
Beautiful. The father would be all right looking
Except his nose is too big. But he
Is smart. He can always answer most things
And when he cannot he says, "Let's look it up," and
Gets a book from their brown library right away
To look it up in, even in the middle of dinner
When the maid is just passing him the platter.
He never says anything nice about
The mother, even when she wears her earrings.
Except once when he and his children were
Looking out the window to see when she
Would come home he saw her in the distance
And they said, "How do you know it's her?"
Because she was still too far away to tell,
And he said, "I know her walk." That
Is as near saying something good about her
As he ever has. The lights really turn on
And off. If I thought it would help, I would ask for a new
Father for Christmas, but they come in pairs and what
Would I do with the new mother? Maybe she could be
A governess. But I do not know if the new father
Would be any different. There is a loaf of bread
In the bread box and red celluloid flames in the fireplace.

TRANSFER

Wind spiked the points of branches into the gray
And swung the wires against it.
Trees and wires cracked the sky and were the cracks
In the gray skin.
Any minute someone from that children's story
Would run through the crumpled field below
The window, yelling or crowing—
Whatever a talking chicken does—
Warning us to run for safety, but giving no direction.

I am tired. I did not sleep, but sat
By the window all night, prepared in case it happened.
The fissures glowed like lava streams
Against the dark. I was afraid
The sun would reveal something I could not imagine.

Now, in the new light, I find only
The healed sky, pink as proudflesh.
The wires hang. The trees perform
Their winter function of standing. The cracks are gone.
The chicken about to scream will not come. Calm
Invades the room. I yawn.
In the palm of my right hand are branching cracks,
The print of yesterday's sky. Through the fissures
I look at the subdermal fat tunneled with veins.

UNCOVERING

Today I rejoice; I even treat myself kindly
Because I have uncovered a crucial self-secret:
The reason for my defective memory, the why of my forgetting
Mozart's century or Grinkard's theorem or how to spell
Grinkard or why my Grandfather left Houston in disgrace
Or whose ear precipitated whichever war it was or more
Of Mending Wall than, "Something there is that doesn't love a wall,"
Or what's that painter's name I met three times this fall, the one
With the red beard or where did the electric company say
To send the letter of complaint about the bill?

What a relief to know
It is not because I never learned self-discipline
By doing my Latin the way Delight Tolles told me I should.
It is not because I gave my roommate cat ringworm
And did not even punish myself by catching it.
It is not because I love chocolate and pâté de foie gras with truffles
Or dislike summer squash and tucked it under the side
Of my plate at camp instead of eating it three times a week.
It is not because my mother would not buy me the dress with ruffles
I needed to prove I was definitely a girl.
It is not because I never learned to sing triplets
Accurately and therefore had to cheat whenever I sang *Ballo*.
It is not because I touched myself in the wrong places
And did not get black circles the way my mother said I would.
It is not because my first reader had only blue and orange pictures.
It is not because I flushed my sister's guppies down the toilet
And convinced the governess she had done it herself.
It is not because I had a governess.
It is not because neither my sister nor I had guppies
And I talk as if we did.
It is not because I tied the door of my son's bedroom when he was two

So he could not wander the house at night,
Even though I had been horrified when Gesell
And Ilg said that was the right thing to do.
It is not because a bee got into my sandal when I was on the swing
Or because termites got into my head through my ears.
It is not because my mother could not sing.
It is not because the house in California was made of brick
Stuck together with fear.
It is not because Jane Flauren lied to Leslie Chabay about me.
It is not because I was born on Ground Hog Day and the ground hog
Went back into his hole and got stuck there.
It is not because the house in Rye was too damp.
It is not because I three times forgot to meet Aunt Leila for lunch
Even though she helped pay for my camp.
It is not because I did not admit at my deflowering
That I was a virgin because I was so embarrassed at being
A still-perfect flower at twenty-three.
It is not because I so often ruffled my father's hair
Which made him scream with temper.
It is not because I hated my father.
It is not because my father took me to see Sonja Henie make a movie.
It is not because I loved my father.
It is not because I went for a walk
And lay in the snow to watch Richard Wharton and
Lisa Gottbaum sit in his living room
And talk.
It is not because I told my shrink lies about why
I could not keep appointments and truths I wish I hadn't.
It is not because the sky is falling down.

I am flooded with relief: it is none of the above.
It is because of a chemical dissolving cells

Inside my skull, hexing me with its hex, enough
Says the Pure Food and Drug Administration to damage
The brain if used regularly as I have for twenty years:
Phisohex.

COUPLING

We are not conceited,
Not at all like those couples who marry
Images of themselves; so when you try to say
The baby looks just like . . .
You realize just like both.
We're completely different:
We won't ever look alike however many
Years we gnarl and wrinkle together
And face each other's faces. Unlike
Inside too, but sitting here
Under this tree which makes a sky of
White flowers over us
I lose my ability to enumerate
And trace the outline of your mouth
With my finger. We make love
On the spread-out Sunday *Times*
Because the ground is wet
And afterwards find semen on the President's face.

II

SUMMER LETTER / SHELL SEKIYU

Do I like Japan, you ask, and to answer with persimmons
Drying, stone gardens, blue roof tiles, would be unfair.
These delights do not make up for the jostlers spoiling
Every walk, or the drivers all breast-fed on kamikaze,
Proceeding as if at midnight east of Minidoka, Idaho,
Not in the cram of noontime Tokyo (Azabu district).

So as I drive I think of your question, and raging
At the truck coming at me—in my lane but certain
I will stop—cursing at the cyclist spurting past my left
As I attempt a left turn, at the taxi's pincer tactics,
I say I hate the Japanese, who are Japan . . . would smash
The truck head-on, smash the grinning face behind the glass
If I could, and not be caught. I dream of buying a tank
And advancing, righteously armored, to crush them all.

Tokyo is mostly a fury decorated with interest,
Ugly, ludicrous, menacing—like a porcupine
(Do they have porcupines in Japan? I'll ask):
Perhaps a gentle heart beats beneath the barbs
And order sings beneath the quills. One would need
To be a taxidermist to know. Right now, though,

I park the car in an alley to write my fury down,
To let it boil until, first a rattle, then a whine,
The valve is pushed up, steam escapes, the pressure
Falls and the explosive act—the damage—is averted.
I sit here in my Toyopet Crown writing, and a boy
Walks by, giggles, looks at the car and giggles again.
Giggles: why? I get out. Greenish-white foam gushes
Through the grille. I stare. Will it explode? Turn off
The engine or leave it running? I stand beside my Toyopet
Erupting, transfixed as the Pompeiians must have been.

A three-wheeled truck in a hurry (all the trucks here
Are in hurries) comes down the road, turns into the alley,
Stops. The driver looks out. Grins. "No danger, no
Danger," he says, waves his hands to reassure me.
"*Matte, matte*" and points. Wait. "*O-mizu*" which must be
The radiator. Turns away. "*Matte, matte*" his words trail
Behind. At the gate of the nearest house, rings the bell.
No answer. Rings again, walks to the back. No answer.

He returns, "*Matte*" and goes to the next house, hidden
Behind a wall. The gate is locked. Rings: no answer.
Another house: the door is opened, and after the bows—
He bows, she bows, they bow—points to me and explains.
Returns with a blue plastic pail. *O-mizu.* Uncaps
The radiator, and Fuji erupts again. Fills it with water,
Then returns the bucket. The bows conjugated again.

I thank him: "*Domo arrigato gozaimashita*" but
He is not finished. He starts the car, revs the motor,
Wipes the seat before I replace him on it. I offer:
"For your time, small presento?" He refuses, gravely.
Then come the bows—rather he bows, I nod. Meanwhile
We have cooled off, the Toyopet and I. It does not
Like the heat, nor do I, as you know. So this autumn
When we are all eating the dried persimmons—they are
Bitter and I do not know why we like them so much—
Or even this winter when snow which is infrequent here
Blurs the stone gardens a little, I will write again.

FALL LETTER / Shell Sekiyu

It is cooler and we are taking our first trip, the four of us
And the Ohtas, Mac's old Japanese friends. We left Tokyo
At 8 A.M. The train ride was uneventful, except at Atami where,
When the train stopped, Mac and Mr. Ohta got off to get
A special kind of obento: eel, rice and cabbage pickle
Arranged in a box made of wood thin as a model plane's wings.
While they were debating about which one of the arrangements
To choose, the train almost left without them. It is hard
To realize how briefly it stops. No more than two minutes.

Now we are on a bus (the only foreigners) on the way
From Shuzenji to Toi. I cannot believe it is so beautiful
After the ugliness of Tokyo where beauty is hoarded,
A private possession to be shared sparingly as dried fish
During the war. Ohta-San says he stood in line
For five hours and when he reached the counter
They grabbed his arm and gave him a typhus shot instead
Of fish. He is beside me now as the bus speeds along
A mountain road, which makes the road through Loveland Pass—
The one where you and I put snow in the radiator when the car
Boiled over—look straight and wide. This one is single lane
With a sheer drop on one side. The vegetation seems tropical
In its abundance, although, as you know, I am no botanist.

Giant white lilies with orange tongues in them lean over
The road. Springing grass races in green waterfalls
Down the banks. Something like laurel explodes in dark
Stars above, and from below a kind of tree I've never
Seen arches up and over. Its huge leaves, each with six
Sharp fingers, reach. Fronds, sprays, vines, branches
Reach and arch. I blink. The branches are hung with
Yellow monkeys, chattering and shooting, live fruit of

23

Nineteen-forty-three movies, my childhood introduction
To Japan. (You would be amazed that war films like
The Halls of Montezuma and *Bridge on the River Kwai*
Are popular here. *The Star Spangled Banner* is played
As incidental music between shows. One time, the children
Stood up, blondly conspicuous. Fragments pierced my back
As candy bars became grenades, the projector a mortar.)
I blink again. The bus rushes through the green tunnel.

We are stopping. A truck faces us. We are in the crotch
Of the zig of a zig-zag. Our girl conductress smiles
And holds up her hand. "*Chotto matte, kudasi.*" Before
Ohta-San speaks we understand . . . "Please wait a minute."
She is getting out and going behind the bus. We hear her
Blow a whistle in short, even bursts. The bus is
Backing up. Ohta-San explains: the driver cannot see
The edge; so she blows and he backs until she stops.
My God, if she sneezes! Please tell Mother we would like
To be cremated here; I'm sure it is cheaper. And tell
Her to see if one of the big hospitals in Tokyo or even
Osaka has corneal transplant facilities so they can use
My eyes for the blind. The company will help her inquire.

We are starting forward again. No sneeze. We have planned
To go to Kyoto this winter, a time when tourists are absent.
I will write then, or perhaps before, if another Z or S
Does not transform the trip into a permanent fall.

Workmen are here packing our belongings. They are putting
Everything in crates which they construct in the living room.
They—the crates—are so beautiful I think
We will not unpack them when we get home.

We leave next week and I am glad, tired of living
Small town life—the town of foreigners—within the biggest
City in the world (or is that London?). One is outside of life,
Looking, responding, being looked at. My poems move more and more
Toward quaint attenuations: Amy Lowell at her weakest.
I have a batch I could call *Tales of Tengenjii*, Tengenjii being
The trolley stop nearest our house, the reference point to use
For Japanese who need directions (addresses mean nothing here
And street names, provided by the Government for major streets
Before the 1964 Olympics, are only used by foreigners).
The title is not bad; only the poems are. One of the best:

> Sitting in my Tokyo house, I turn
> the radio on; shrunk small by a bonsai people,
> it sings Aida in a tumult of Italian sound.

> Tunnel straight through the world,
> starting at Times Square and you *will*
> be upside down when you come out,
> alone, round-eyed, smelling of meat.

> O patria mia, O America
> I am lonely;
> I long . . .
> Rivedro le foreste imbalsamate

> I hold the Sony close to my body,
> my static-filled love partner.

I guess I have discovered I do not transplant well. Imagine that
You have lived in a Burton Holmes Travelogue for over a year
And you will understand why I am glad to be leaving. As the sun
Sinks slowly in the West—yes, even here—we bid farewell, etc.

III

THE INSIDE STORY

Elsie sat, reading *The Cat in the Hat,*
Analyzing its rhyme scheme.
The cellar flooded. Elsie put Chopin
On the record player and turned the volume higher.

The house caught on fire;
It was completely burned.
Elsie moved the family to an apartment and painted
The flames, calling the picture "Winter Overturned."

Her husband, because she ignored him,
Developed a series of psychosomatic ailments.
She painted his portrait, complete with boils,
In oils.

When her children turned to slate,
She realized what she had done,
But although she sang to them and painted
Their gray bodies flesh pink,
They remained stone.

A FAMILY QUESTION

Dear Dr.
Franzblau, I have
A problem, or perhaps I should say
Problems. To begin at the beginning: I have no information
About myself until I was born: a ten-month, sixteen-pound baby.
My mother who was rather small was never the same again. We
Had been Catholics—that is why they left me
In so long, sacredness of unborn life,
Etc.—but when my Ma gained sufficient
Strength she shaved her head
And became a Hasidic Jew.

The first months
Of my life I was neglected.
Poor mother was too weak to attend
To me, none of my three sisters was old enough
And Father did not take over for Ma; he hated babies,
Children, too, and was seldom home, especially as for certain
Medical reasons which I needn't spell out for you, Doctor,
My mother was no longer available to him. She never
Was again. Even after her health would have
Permitted, she said her religion
Would not allow a Catholic
To be the father of
Her children.

My childhood
Was also less than usually
Happy. We were all bedwetters and
In those days we had no washing machines. There was
Enough to eat, but it was always Brussels sprouts, Brussels
Sprouts. The big time of the week at our house was Friday afternoon

When whoever had been good got to shave Ma's head. The sister
Right above me—eleven months older—was a pyrotechniac.
She lit fires. Reform school, then jail; we gradually
Lost track of her. Even today when I read
That the origin of a fire is unknown,
I wonder if it could be
Dear, old Mag.

So when I say,
Keeping in mind my background,
As I know you will, that I think I did pretty well
To finish school and get a job as mail girl with the Shell
Oil Co.—Blue Cross, paid vacations, three weeks after five
Years, a pension plan, etc.—I think you might agree.
It was on one of those vacations, a singles week
In Pennsylvania Dutchland, that I met Harry.
He was really great: good-looking, neat
And had a good job.

It's the old story.
If I knew then what I know now,
But I didn't, not even for almost a year after
We were married. How can I put it? After awhile
He didn't want to do it unless I did it with other men
And told him about it. Sometimes I went along, but I never really
Wanted to. And when I won't he gets furious and picks
A fight over nothing. Like, because I can't broil meat,
The smell reminds me too much of dear, old Mag,
He'll yell at me and say he only likes meat
Broiled and every other way is lousy. So,
Dr. Franzblau, I hope I've given you
Enough to go on. Yours
Truly, Troubled

Dear Troubled,
Yes, your information
Has been most helpful. There are two things
You must do to get your marriage
On a solid footing.

First, find
Yourself a hobby. You are currently
Too absorbed in yourself and your problems.
As an example of how a hobby could help you, suppose
You take up decoupage. Then when your husband yells at you
About the meat, you can be planning how to trim
Your next box—a figure from Godey's Ladies
Book, perhaps, with just a touch of gold
Lace trim—until the storm
Is over.

Second, you must
Learn how your unconscious
Antipathy to men—generated way back when your
Father refused to, figuratively, suckle you—is
Probably causing your husband to act out the role-confusion you
Impose on him. As he is using you as an intermediary in homosexual
Fantasies, your becoming aware of how such confusion
Operates must ultimately affect his behavior.
Awareness and the willingness
You have shown to seek help by
Consulting me are the first
Steps on the road to change.
Good luck, Dr. Rose
Franzblau

The poet told me if I was serious
I must isolate myself for at least a year—
Not become a hermit, but leave
My family, job, friends—so I did. My sister
Agreed to take over as mother though not
As wife. I wonder if she will become that too;
I've always thought maybe she didn't marry
Because she wanted Howard herself. So I
Have moved here to North Dakota where
I work in a gas station, the only woman s.s.
Attendant in N.D. Nowhere could be more isolated
And no job could: whistles and "baby
Pump some of that to me" crack in the cold
Or melt in the summer.

       try   try   try
    crycry   crycry   crycry   cry

I have been here seven months. Poetry should
Be flowing from my navel by now, if . . .
Out of the solitude, I expected I would erect
Something magnificent, the feminine analogue
Of Jeffer's tower. Maybe it would have gone
Into the ground instead of up.

   s   k   y
                       high

I have discovered I drink when I am solitary. I
Have discovered I can read page ninety-two of
Remembrance of Things Past twenty times in solitary
Without ever reading it. If I don't die of alcoholism,
I will of cholesterol: solitary cooking.

fryfryfry   fryfry   fryfryfryfry   frydie

Rhyme is important, my way of keeping
A grip on things. I wonder if the poet meant
It would all happen after I left, or if he is a sadist
Who wants to send all those stupid enough to sit
At his feet to N.D. or S.D. or West Va.,
Hazing before possible joining. I wonder if Jean
Is in the double bed.

                tower

                power

I cannot think about the children, but I
Do all the time. "Women artists fail
Because they have babies." The last thing I wrote
Was "The Children at the Beach" and that was over
A month ago. I am alone so I have to have company so
I turn on TV; at home
I only turned it off.

           thumbtacks   processionals
                  north
                   red

It is time to go to work. First I need a drink. I consider
The Smirnoff bottle on the coffee table; a fly
Lands on it. And then it all happens: the life
Of that bottle flashes before me. Little by little,
Or quickly, it is used up; empty, as clear as it was
Full, it journeys to the dump; it rests upon the mounds of
Beautiful excess where what we are—

Sunflowers, grass, sand—
Is joined to what we make—
Cans, tires and it itself in every form of bottle.
I put on my s.s. coveralls, a saffron robe, knowing I have found
What I was sent to find. The sky speaks to me; the sound
Of the cars on Highway 2 is a song. Soon I will see the pumps,
Those curved rectangles shaped like the U.S. and smell the gas,
Our incense. O country, O moon, O stars,
O american rhyme is yours is mine is ours.

RICHARD'S BOOK AND CHOPPER GANZ

for Richard Elman

We have read the above manuscript as requested. There is a serious problem because the author's parents, a principal subject of this book, are mocked and held up to contempt and made to seem unfit as parents if not dreadful people as well. Accordingly, Baffin Books should obtain a written release from the author's parents before publication may be considered.

> Gans means goose and ganz means
> Everything, quite, entirely.
> The radio announcer slurs the name
> So it is unclear whether to think of him
> As goose or, in this case, gander
> Or as everything, quite, entirely which
> Is more appropriate because on November tenth
> He thoroughly killed his parents with
> A Boy Scout axe. "Be prepared," and he was.
> Or is that the motto for geese?

In addition we have the following specific comments:

Page 6—The incident in which the author's brother dangled him from the 12th floor of an apartment building by the feet is libelous and should be deleted unless it may be proven true or a release obtained from the brother.

Page 26—The reference to Mrs. Mullaney's "funky heavy menstrual smell" could be libelous and could be an invasion of privacy in some states. Accordingly, it should be deleted or the identification changed so that Mrs. Mullaney is no longer identifiable.

I do not know the details of the murders,
Whether he minced them into choplets and droplets
And stored the pieces in jars. Or whether
He simply severed enough to complete
The execution. Or whether he danced and
Whirled and spatter-painted the room with blood
And screamed with the joy of creating.

Page 31—The reference to Vera Scheep's private parts could be an invasion of privacy in some states. Accordingly, it should be deleted unless all the identifying details have been changed so that she is not identifiable.

Page 34—Same general comment as stated above with regard to the author's parents as applied to the statement that they were "a household of psychopaths."

He had only been out of Bellevue (where
The radio says he had been taken after
Eccentric behavior had been observed)
For a week. His craziness was not the fury,
But the axe. That at thirty the only way
He could leave home was to hack his way out.

Page 90—The portrait of the author's teacher, Daniel Curley, would be an invasion of privacy in some states. It may also be libelous in that he is described as "the ugliest looking person I had ever seen . . . an anjou pear gone rotten." It should be deleted unless all identifying details have been changed so that Curley is not identifiable.

Page 131—The reference to Roger Kornfeld as a "moron" and his parents as "another set of monsters" is libelous and should be deleted

unless all the identifying details of all parties have been changed so
that they are no longer identifiable.

> Poor Ganz, has he proved that he is crazy
> Now that he no longer is, now that
> He has deleted the source of his craziness
> And changed the identifying details so
> That his parents are no longer identifiable.

REPLY TO THE REQUEST FROM THE
REMAINING POET FOR
SUICIDE SUGGESTIONS

I shall not spend time on the alternatives of living,
But shall, as you requested, suggest fresh ways of leaving life.
Reading between the lines of your letter,
Which I must say was difficult to read at all,
Blotched as it was with red and yellow stains (did one
Of Dorothea's children spill the trifle on it?), I think
You are consulting me not so much for a checklist
Of unused methods which would distinguish your death
From that of your immediate colleagues and friends (I am sure
You have already ruled out a bridge, a gun, a walk
Before a car) as for a whole new vocabulary of dying.
I have given the matter much thought (in fact I stayed home
Last night from *Götterdämmerung*, for which I had
Already purchased tickets, to think it through).
Three plans asserted themselves sufficiently often
For me to pay them serious attention: I have selected
One which I will save for last, the best for last. (Interesting
That dessert intrudes again, but perhaps a suicide so planned as
That we speak of is life's Baked Alaska.) However,
First I shall describe the two rejected, in case you wish alternatives.

1) You buy a sailing vessel, like Chichester,
And let excitement build about your trip around the world.
The press must be informed that all you know of sailing was learned
The summer you were seven and almost drowned
Off Falmouth. It is your lack of seamanship which makes
Your solo trip unique. You get yourself
Well out to ocean (you may need to arrange a tow
For this in order not to founder in sight of shore and other boats),

39

Then drenched in a magnificat of blue which
Sea and sky provide (assuming the day is fine),
Tack the manuscript of your suicide poems to the mast
And wait. Or slip overboard if slow deaths
Do not appeal to you. (You did not make this clear
In your letter. In fact, you really gave me insufficient guidance.)
The strength of this method seems to me to lie
In its metaphor. The weaknesses are two: the dying
Could be painful (again, I lack your guidance) or the boat
Could capsize before being found, making
Your death look accidental. The latter problem might be
Partially overcome by installing a ship-to-shore radio in the vessel
And, after requesting a good stenographer, reading
The poems over it. However, again there are two disadvantages
To this sub-plan: You might be rescued against your will. Your will
Might weaken and the radio would let you change your course.

2) You could enlist in the war we have so long decried
And get yourself killed, preferably by the South Vietnamese.
The strength of this plan is it turns your death into a protest,
But that is also its weakness. Assuming
You have managed to convince the Marines of the reviving
Qualities of verse and they have appointed you a poet-medic
And you are in Vietnam, words dripping
Through the tubes instead of blood and the appropriate
Moment for getting shot presents itself and you quickly put on
Clothing with Viet Cong markings and *do*
Get shot, if you acknowledge it is suicide for reasons
Other than the war it is not protest and if
It is not both, the method seems too cumbersome to be worthwhile.
(The news of James Wright's latest award from
The Academy of American Poets was put on the obituary page

Of The N.Y. Times so perhaps even America's leading newspaper
Has our sense of the poet's occupation as fatal.)

3) *My favorite.* You assemble in the great hall
Of that baronial hulk you are renting: Dorothea, her children
By Adleburt and Fitzhugh-Dickingson, Andrew (in the picture
You sent he looks just like you, but with Dorothea's
Pointed chin) and, if possible, Sarah (I remember her
At Andrew's age. She looked like Phyllis, but
Clearly had your nose). I realize Phyllis may not
Permit Sarah to rush across the Atlantic during the school year,
But perhaps she can convince her mother. Of course, if
You can get Phyllis to come, too, and somehow get her to agree
To participate (the mind boggles—not only your children
By both women and two sets of steps, but both women as well . . .)
Anyway, you get as many as you can into the great hall,
Seating them in tiers as for an old fashioned photograph.
You have the camera placed beforehand, focused, etc. with
Its time-lapse gadget set to allow you to get into
The picture after pressing the button. I have sent you today,
Air freight, a Hasselblatt portrait camera with double-synchronized
Flashbulbs. One, untampered with, will give the flash.
The other, filled by me with gelignite, will do just that:
Ignite into explosion. The fuse is in the shutter-trip device.
I have included extra bulbs and fuse cords though I am certain
Only one set will be needed. After pressing
The button you assume your place in the center.
When the flash illumines the family group, death will occur
Instantaneously, that is within seconds, for all in the room.
(Be sure Nanny is not allowed in.) Somehow I feel
This one is right for you. It includes the family, as your work
So often has, destroys it, as your work has attempted

41

But has not fully realized, and, paradoxically, preserves it.
The method of dispatch is neat, fool-proof (the failed suicide is
Foolish) and quite special. In a time when news without
A photograph is incomplete, the manner of your death will be
Complete, something none of those you are linked with
Could have claimed. Be sure your volumes are next to your chair
And that you are holding one, with the title visible,
At the time of the flash. Please leave instructions
To have one of the photographs sent to me. I shall look at
It often with affection and, yes, a certain amount of pride.

IV

RIDDLE

He is doing to her what I am doing to him;
She does not know what he is doing to her;
And he does not know what I am doing to him.
She and he are both taller than I am.
She is open, he is hiding, I am hidden.
P. is blue-eyed, B. is double-jointed, F.
Has a generous mouth. None of the Indians
Can ride in a boat with a cannibal. I am
The only one of the three who knows
That he is doing to her what I am doing to him.
Question: Who is an Indian and who is a cannibal?

EIGHT FOR LUNCHEON

The guests arrived at quarter past twelve that May afternoon,
    A perfect blue and green day. The day's
    Perfection pleased me because I *do* prefer
    To display my birds against a ground of
    Foliage and sky which matches them.
At luncheon, al fresco, the man with the curly brown beard
    Amused us over the gazpacho with his puns.
    Conversation during the omelette aux fines herbes
    Centered around the political scene, dominated
    By the other—salt and pepper—bearded man.
The black woman smiled occasionally, just enough to let us know
    She understood the language. After coffee,
    I rose and led them to the weeping beech. (I
    Had placed the cages there before the guests had
    Come. The huge tree with its dome of branches
Curving to the ground forms a natural enclosure which I think is
    Fitting for the beauty of my birds.) When
    The guests had had a chance to see each bird
    Within its cage, I let them out, one by one.
    They posed, perching on the wrought-gold
Finials of their cages or on the lower branches of the tree:
    Turquoise, indigo, orange flecked with yellow,
    Scarlet, beetle green and past the colors
    Of imagination. The brown curly bearded man
    Took a sling shot from his pocket and hit
The purple-crested cockatoo mid-wattle. He was less than
    Ten feet from the bird; so little shooting
    Skill was needed. Several of the others
    Found, or had brought, their own weapons:
    Rocks, sticks, stilettos, tiny beebee guns.
They opened fire or stabbed or threw until the ground was bright
    With feathers. The non-participants in the kill

Watched, looking questions, but not speaking them.
Then the man with the brown beard consulted his
Watch and said he had another engagement. The others
Consulted their watches, too, thanked me for a delightful time
And left. I picked up the bodies—birds look
Unbelievably small without their feathers—and
Returned them to their cages. I really had not
Known until that afternoon the way the others felt.

BREAKING SEALS

Even when I was only six I became aware of the talent
I had for working with seals. I trained them
To come to me when I whistled. They nuzzled their noses
Through the iron railing surrounding their pond
At the Central Park Zoo and nibbled my braids.

Now I am Esmerelda, the Seal Lady Wizard, star
Of the Circus Maroni. My seals tightrope walk,
Ride elephants, sell popcorn. They are truly astounding.
I am known here and there as the greatest seal trainer.

But I despair and must punish myself. I rend
Cascades of tissue paper till it covers the floor and
My bed, rustling me awake night after night.
I oversalt my soup and permit myself few sips of water,
Condemning myself to interior oceans. I spend months
Carving sculptures of soap which I place in the toilet.
These torments I earn by my pretense,
The pretense of being an expert seal trainer.

Lovely, slippery emblems of my skill: I know my own
Ineptitude with you, no matter what the world thinks.
I will never get you to sing the sextet from *Lucia*,
To recite the Ten Commandments, to keep your elbows
Off the table. I cannot admit that I do not know all
That there is to know about you. I can only confide
My ignorance to you because seals do not have ears.

GUIDE TO THE RUNES

for Richard Howard

Water seeps into the house
through hidden cracks;
    water finds the cracks
the way
        wasps can. She
enjoys the moisture—
it has been a dry
        winter—but there
is too much: the encyclopedia
has to be moved to
    a higher shelf.

The plumber says he'll
    come

The guide's head is reflectively bald; he has no memorized spiel
But follows the rules formulated beneath his too-evident skull.
The patterns he celebrates are not ritual by rote; they repeat because
Pattern is repetition and revealing order, the function of guides.

But doesn't, and is
    the plumber the one?
        Or the mason?
            Or Noah?
Not Noah; forty days
    and forty nights
            coupled;
things are too
        fluid.

So, that describes his function, but how does he accomplish the job?
He cannot be called guide if he does not guide; so describe
The guided. They are confused and annoyed, wanting the tape-recorded
Message about the bathroom fixtures at Versailles, instead
Of his instruction that, before they can even begin to climb the hill,
They must first examine the eighteenth-century garden where he will
Reveal the topiary trees—spiders and bees—and show them the grotto
Embedded with tusks and horns won by the poet in animal lotto.

She sits letting the water
　　　　rise
around her. Death
　　by inundation.
　　　　They will all cry.
Flowers in her hair: Ophelia.
　　　　She splashes
　　　　　　across the room
to get the available flowers,
straw,
　　　to have them ready.

　　　What she has
made,
　　all that is most

To distract his way and have theirs, they say they are hungry, the Electro-media
Luncheonette is in the next block and a light lunch would make his encyclopedia
More digestible . . . or even brown rice and herbs at the tearoom of Honganji
　　　　　　　　　　　　　　　　　　　　　　　temple,

Where the cashier is an abacist and the gardens are black and white stones, would
　　　　　　　　　　　　　　　　　　　　be acceptable.

But, he, recognizing ruse as well as he does spells and runes,
Says, "We will continue. On your left is a birch disguised as blue spruce."

important to her,

will float

up (along

with her body

and other

household

flotsam)

and will be found and

dried

and read:

an uncomfortable way to

gain

attention.

She tries to compose

a final

especially meaningful

page, but

Row, row, row your boat

circulates through her

head

instead.

The group is becoming tired, uncomfortably pruned like the trees, by his words
which slice

At their complacencies. "Where's the rest room?" "We will rest at the top." He
moves toward the base

Describing the climb: "Almost ninety thousand identical steps to the summit,
A systematic construction which must be systematically mounted;
So as the first part of a circular route this group will ascend the ninety thousand
Steps." "But circling up and down is impossible without going underground."
"Like you, a circle subverts direction." They are furious, call him prick-eared,
But he is immune to insult from the guided and insists on the indefinite sphere.

She sits
        waiting;
            the water rises;
each time it reaches her
        mouth
            she has to
move
            up; drowning
                in a room
    is not
            like turning
                on the gas. She

climbs
on a chair
 then
on the bridge table to
 breathe.
Breathing is stronger
 than
 decision.

They start the climb. He guides, leading or prodding from behind.
The sun illuminates the crevices which he points out, emphasizing they were
 planned

By the water which is the crevice-maker, however much another maker
Claims water skills. "This is not what we paid for. You are a faker.
We won't continue. We could, but you are unfit; we want a refund."
He starts to order them on, but they cannot continue; they lie on the ground,
Their feet worn off, like fingers of lepers in the leprosorium band.
He has stuffed their ears with conundrums, overdazzled their eyes: they are deaf
 and blind.

Only birds, the hierarch, his head reflecting sun, and the strongest two
Of the group are left. They turn from crevice blood and eyes blank as grapes to
 continue.

54

The table collapses;

she
    inhales water
    fast
to hurry death
       and out
       and in
    she is underwater
       and breathing.

Gills? No
       gills.

She moves in slow water time
doubting her breathing
       and breathing.

They have almost reached the top, completing one-quarter of the circle, but
Night is coming and the guide agrees they must stop soon. Birds, treeless, roost
On their shoulders. Caught in the transition between seeing and having to feel,
       they pun

To ward off *anomia*. The anti-twilight arch mirrors the fading sun
And the steps are evening distinct 'in a light committed to impartiality,'
But they sit as if it is no longer possible to see. The reality

Of darkness is accepted, even insisted upon, before it is dark.
The guide strokes the bird housed on his shoulder and sings, "Ark, Ark the Lark."

Drowning has failed.
She
will leave.
The door knobs
will not
turn,
nothing will open
or break.

Delivery men
come to the door
occasionally
but they do not see her
however
wildly
She gesticulates or
calls. She looks
out the
window wondering who
will deliver her. How?
And for what?

The sun shines on
the blue
hyacinths—is that
a translation from the French?
She touches
the glass, pretending
she can feel
the April
air.

In the morning, if they get to the top, the air at the edge will be
A mirror, making the half from the quarter. The two, expecting to see
The revelation promised by the brochure will see themselves and will turn
Back. The guide will continue the last few steps prepared for the join
Of mirror and rock where the reflection is always closer to the edge than he,
Reminding him each trip that image is more perilous than actuality.
This time instead of the mirrored duplicate he will find clear glass
And beyond it, the confusion of clarity. A woman facing him gesticulates as
If under water. He cannot lip-read yet, but will hurry down the slope
Illuminated with possibility. After buying a manual for the deaf, he will pick up
                    his next tour group.

AL FRIED

Alfried—really Alfred Fried, but the kids ran his name into one
Like Siegfried—got terrible colds each September. His mother
Put him in warm pyjamas—even when it was hot
As it always was for the Jewish holidays during which he atoned
With double sweats, caused by flannel on top of fever—and fed him
Turkey soup because she was an original, unstereotyped,
At least in regard to soup, Jewish mother. How could it be
That he, he the pride of the family, the first son could
Want to stay away from school, could catch cold and even
One year develop it into pneumonia to avoid that place of good things.
Now he knows that that's what the colds were. He sits at the table
And tells me that that's what they were. He teaches at the College,
Has just published his second book and has even been
Written up in the Public Affairs section of Newsweek. We talk;
He blows his nose and opens a package of Pine Bros. honey drops.
It is September.

PAST ORDERING

Driving through March 6th alone in the fog,
Even sounds are absent as if damped by felts.
The trees lining the road fence the edge of a flat world.
Any minute I expect Onegin and Lenski, with seconds,
To walk between blurred hedges ready to fight their dawn duel
While expressionless Tatjana sings:
Oh, help from Above for my love, for my love I am burning.
Yes, there they are in that field, pacing the steps apart,
Then turning.

It is only the Hunt Club yard men pushing wheelbarrows of manure
Which they will sell. Manure is precious:
The onion farmers failed for lack of it when horses were replaced
By cars.

Oblivious of the manure, Lenski turns at the count to shoot.
He demanded satisfaction—and he gets it . . . up on the toes,
Pause . . . Clutch . . . Fall . . . The tenor has been upset.

Suddenly, the rear of a moving van fills the visible space ahead.
I follow the truck's wake, singing with dramatic emphasis:
Though I should die for it, I swear that
I first shall sa-a-ti-is-fy my longing . . .
The truck's turn arrow blinks 'right'; I move left
To avoid the wide-swinging rear; when it stops.
I just miss it. Passing, I prepare to give the driver
The up yours sign. His hand on the steering wheel: black,
Then his black face. Now I cannot allow myself to hate him.

The serfs picked berries and sang as Tatjana and Olga
Sat sewing in the garden. The serfs were told to sing
To make sure they didn't eat the berries.

I would like to have given such orders and sent the one
Who disturbed my ride
To Siberia.

ASPECTS OF UNICORNS

I have told you about the unicorns in my dreams,
Embroidered filigree blankets for them, given them
Shoes and elaborate umbrellas, even ear trumpets in case
Their ears are blocked. The creatures live,
But I do not. Talking, talking.

I have ground their horns to powder—the most
Powerful aphrodisiac known to man—and administered
It to my friends. They do not respond, though some
Break out in hives. Talking, talking.

I have butchered them and invited guests to share
The meat and served it skewered on its horn
On a platter on my head, dancing before them naked.
They see the scars of my mastectomy for the first time
And cover the meat with catsup and pineapple. Talking, talking.

I gave the unicorns everything precious, but they
Did not notice. I slaughtered them and used them as bribes;
They proved ineffectual. Yet I must use them.
The umbrella blows inside out and one of its ribs
Pierces mine. It is the unicorn's horn.
It is not. I can still tell umbrellas and unicorns
Apart. Talking, talking.

PAINTINGS FROM THE SLAUGHTER HOUSE:
A SLIDE SHOW OF HOGS

This is a quick sketch: at first there was only about
Two minutes to catch each hog, to render it.
I tried to get the details of a hoof, a head,
The mammary glands as they went past. (Next slide, please.)
Two pigs, snout by snout, an interesting balance
Of flesh, curves and holes . . . It was so slippery—
Blood—that I had trouble with my footing.

> He wears a black Bulgarian suit
> To paint in, carries blood secrets
> In his lunch box and his
> Paints in a brown Jocasta bag.
> (The slaughterhouse has no cafeteria.)

After a week or so, I relaxed and began to relate
To the hogs. You can see the warmer quality.
(Next) An interesting perspective: the head
Below me and the hind legs stretching up
To where the steel hooks pierce them.

> His mother is always sick,
> Calling for him, moaning his
> Name through bubbles of saliva
> Which make him think that she
> Is dying. She has survived many deaths.
> (He is not an employee, therefore ineligible for Blue Cross.)

These took longer, up to six minutes; time I gained
By following the subject pig around the moving circle of
The conveyor track on which it hung. After a while

The workers got to know me and sometimes slowed the track.
(Next) Some critics haven't liked the reds
I used to catch this sow in oil on paper.

> He sits in a field, dreaming
> Of his sister, as he paints
> The flowers: they are his sister's
> Parts. Bees nuzzle her breasts.
> (The slaughterhouse is closed on Sundays.)

But after friendliness, demands on me began. The men
Wanted drawings, not sketches of the parts,
But the entire pig or even groups. They didn't realize
It took perhaps a week to get one that I thought
Was right. (Next) I love the angle
Of the crotch and did a series of them. They have
For me a quality which is voluptuous.

> When he cannot paint, he folds
> Paper into white cranes to bring
> His family better fortune. He has
> Tin boxes filled with cranes
> Stored in his closet.
> (The lard cans are a useful size and come with lids.)

Heads: round-headed pigs, the kind they use
For head cheese. The men were angry when I wouldn't
Give them finished drawings, began to hide the heads
In the machinery. But I discovered how to get some
From the freezer. They were heavy; I embraced them;
An armful, I can tell you (Next). Full-length
Body: some have said it has a quality of Venus.

He casts horoscopes, skewering people
To their stars, telling them what
They are and will become, and
What he is: Leo with Aries rising.
He is dark-haired in his Lion House.
(Yellow helmets are required for everyone within the plant.)

The veterinarian wanted me to draw him beside a hanging
Carcass. When I wouldn't—the hogs were difficult enough
Without injecting humans—he threatened to declare me
A sanitary risk. The fear that I might have to stop
Before the subject was exhausted shows, I think,
As frenzy in the paint (Next), this one (Next)
And this (Next). A melting quality: the pigs
Dissolving in the fire through which they're put to stop the blood
And singe the hair off. You know I am a vegetarian.

He sleeps. The walls of his room
Turn to flame. His mother wakes him
From his screaming and brews
Him garlic tea to ward off evil.
(Albino pig skin is saved for burn skin-grafts.)

Many pigs, more fully drawn and painted. One day
The circling overhead conveyor belt went wild,
Then stopped, releasing them: pigs whirling
Through the air, landing all around us. One crushed
The foreman's leg. I used the time of porcine chaos
To do this group: limb over limb, reds mingling,
Snout merging into snout, body within body, and yet
Each one distinct: a fugue of pigs.

He is lying in the snow, painting it,
Licking it, washing the red from
His pictures with snow, freezing his pulse
Until it slows to a less-painful measure.
He has decided to paint snow scenes.
Occasionally, a little blood throbs in the corner.

THE INSATIABLE BABY

The insatiable baby sucked on its mother.
As the book said, supply increased with demand;
So the baby grew enormously, and
Its anemone-pink mouth fastened to the pink
Bud of her nipple, barnacle to rock.

At six months he grew big as six years, though still
Baby-featured, baby-limbed. One day he swallowed
Her whole right breast, devoured it. But filled
With maternal duty, she gave him her left.

When he had ingested her entire, they built him
A mesh form, towel-covered, with milk and music
Piped in, so he could never-stop. But
The metal milk disagreed: both died,
She inside him, curled like an embryo.

ONE IN A VELVET GOWN

It was a gray day; the dogs were barking.
Big Jill Sprat, née Horner
Sat in a corner, sticking her thumb in
Because she knew she was alone. The plum
Was dark and juicy, but the only man
She had ever loved
Was Jack, not her husband, Jack, but her brother,
Jack, who had sold his stock, left her and town
And gone to London to blow his horn,
While she was left alone with Sprat
Who kept telling her she was overweight,
But ate all the lean and left her
The fat, curds and whey, and pease porridge hot;
So no wonder. The doctor said no wonder
Because she was pregnant, that after nine days
She would deliver from her pot
A bone. Her maternity dress was velvet,
Dark and seductive, but she was alone.
It was a gray day; the dogs were barking.
The beggars were coming to a town of beggars.

REFUSING FURTHER RISK

If there are any offers still outstanding,
I withdraw them
and put notices in all the papers saying so.

My arms kept growing,
trying to reach arrangements :
they extended beyond my ability to manage:
I'd find them half across the room in places I didn't want
them when I woke up. Controlling them used all my time.

Extension is desir-able: there is risk, yes,
but in that risk, possibility flowers until
jungles of color transform geometry, or so I thought
and thought we thought. All that time lost
nurturing malformations. Predictably stunted after the first
as if we'd had retarded children and kept on having them
because we didn't notice or didn't care.

I will not listen to your voice, will never touch you. You try
to hold me to it, threatening or sweet-talking,
but I have learned legalities from you.
Didn't you see my notice; don't you read the papers?
It's too late, too late to ask for it now:
My offer has been withdrawn.

REFLECTIONS IN STONE

I went for stone in the quarry,
Chopping and hacking the lamb-fat blocks
  Into a semblance of order,
I matched the red veins into symmetry.

  What happens when you cover
All the mirrors and then in the mumu
Section of Bloomingdale's you
Discover yourself across the aisle?

The stone arrived today.
Within it, like a cyst, are answers;
  Or, if the cutting is inept,
The knife may reveal metastasized cancer.

  It is you across the aisle,
Not someone resembling you, but you,
From black coat to three moles
On the face and bulges in the same places.

I cut. Diana grown fat
And varicosed emerges from
  My cutting. She was not what I wanted
But she was what I got.

  You wonder if she has noticed
Herself, must catch her eye to find out.
Ask her the time. "I'm sorry,"
She answers, "I never wear a watch."

She was not what I wanted.
United Parcel would not pick

Her up nor could I carve her into shape.
I return to the quarry for another block.

"Time is for the timid":
She holds a pond-blue mumu up
Against her body, looking
At me, reflecting on her image.

But I am afraid to choose more
Stone. The bathtub is filled by one twin,
        There's a single bed in the apartment
And I can't afford to move again.

TWICE TOO LONG

It began as a dwarf but it grew. People
Kept telling the mother it was getting too tall. She only said, What
Can I do? But when it reached six nine although just twelve
           She became alarmed, she became alarmed
And took it to an endocrinologist which was what they had been
                            telling her
To do all along. The doctor said, since female hormones would stop
           The growth but feminize it, too,
The only possible solutions were: compress or amputate. What a
                            choice
For a mother who, no wonder, went, as they say in Paris, completely
           Folle and had to be carted off
To Bellevue when she attempted the amputation herself under the
                            most
Unsanitary conditions, the most unsanitary conditions. It
           Not only continued to grow, it grew
Until it was more than eleven feet and by then they knew it was what
It was and there was no hope of either compressing or amputating . . .
           Therefore, it stands in the corner of
Their living room at two-eight-three Madison Avenue where they
Moved for the high ceilings. And when people say it is too
           Long, it is too long, it chews
Them up and deposits them in the plant-filled Minton jardiniere
                            (where
They make excellent fertilizer). It believes in growing things.

THE HOLY MAN WALKS THROUGH FIRE

They were looking (as they still looked at the flag and
Other residual emblems, feeling a crinkle
Of lost certainties) for someone to show he knew
What they needed. And I, who had three times tried
To kill myself but each time was saved by a quirk,
Decided I was being saved for something. I asked
Myself was I to be the one they looked for?
To answer that question, I applied for grants
From four foundations. Fluent as I am in Yakut,
Chuckchee and Manangkabau—the only man I know of
Fluent in all three—I was able to choose the grant
I chose to analyze how the glottal manipulations
And palate shape of the three tongues affected
The development of their mathematical systems.
I thought I would hurry through my monograph
And spend the time on studying myself. But while
I delved into the rites which ultimately shaped
The tongues which shaped their mathematical
Systems, I found I had found myself before I had looked.

To summarize that initial summary: the man
Who is to lead the village receives a sign
He is being saved from death by a former shaman
Who returns from the bowl of heaven to the plate
Of earth in the guise of an animal. I saw Fred
Breaking the window in his hawk costume the night
Of the Bat Masque as I lay in the gas-filled kitchen.
And then the day I jumped off the ledge and was
Saved from death on the rocks by a blanket of seals.
One large one in particular prevented my shattering.
And finally (and this you can't dismiss as circumstance)
What happened at the third attempt: I tried

To throw myself in front of the A train of the IND.
The train rushed toward me, growing enormously, ready
To meet me. Then, just as I pushed off the edge,
A hand lifted me back, a voice said: Do not fear
The universe. I turned to face my savior, my
Betrayer and saw an almost Oriental, exceptionally tall
For an Oriental, if he was, wearing a blue sweatshirt
Lettered in white: LUMA. Not an animal,
You say? I didn't think so either till,
Examining a Yakut funeral chant, I found
Their shaman's name: Luma, meaning soul-bird.

Once I had deciphered the first meanings
Of the shaman's messages to me, subsequent
Translation accelerated like the breaking
Of a code. I knew now I had been chosen.
But exactly for what and how? The first step,
At any rate, was clear. I discussed mechanics
With the p.r. firm of Schluss and Yamaguchi.
We all agreed that, to save time at the time
When my mission would be revealed,
We should devise a scheme to dramatize
My ability to lead. Techniques which work
In a small settlement, the usual shaman abode,
Cannot be used in country-wide dissemination.

I thought of it myself—I'd walk through fire,
Not just a flaming hoop, but lots.
The p.r. men congratulated me and arranged
To have it televised (prime time) before a studio
Audience. I assured them I had done it many times
Before, which was not true. But I had put myself

74

Through other tests—sleeping in a nest of snakes,
Walking over ice so thin those following fell through.
To fit myself for the ordeal, I read the fire-thought
Of holy men and worked on pain in trance.
I got so that six-inch nails through both
Palms were simply pure white light.

The day came. The Schluss and Yamaguchi ads
Announcing the firewalk had engrossed the nation.
I was assigned my own mailbag, I got so many letters.
They asked advice, sent me money for my cause,
Wrote of love, both physical and spiritual.
I had to disconnect the phone. That afternoon,
Before the walk, I tested my immunity by passing
A deerskin image of myself through the flame
Of my gas stove. It did not burn or even darken;
So I was confident, able to nap before air-time.

The fire was before me, a solid field
Of it, forty by forty feet. I was afraid.
The atmosphere was difficult for trance.
I stared at the TV spots, widening my pupils
Till I soared, a soul-bird. The lights became
The sun, bright, white, dissolving my body,
Moving me through the void into the flame.
It burned. The pain was wordless, beyond
Screaming, telling or retelling. I knew
I could not do it. But I was past the center,
The point of no return.

I have limited
Use of one

. with which
I am writing.
Half the day
I lie on air,
A new technique
Used here to treat
Third-degree
Burn cases. It is
A form of levitation
Worthy of a more
Effective shaman.
The other half
I try to sleep
On sheepskin.
My bones protrude;
My country has not made it through the fire.

DEP

When he cut off his feet I knew he was leaving . . .
A mother's instinct. He sat a moment allowing
The ankle stumps to heal, then walked out the front door.
I didn't try to stop him; I knew he had to go—
Everyone said so. He left me his feet; I
Treasured them because now they had to be all of him.
I felt the toes for messages, crying
Over the corrugated toenails which had always tended
To become ingrown. How many times I had notched
Those nails to ease a swollen corner. I stroked
The skin, touching the rest of his body. I kissed the heels.

He sent me postcards of the Corn Palace, the Mormon Tabernacle,
The Astrodome and Mt. Rainier where he says he
Will stay for a while. I mounted the cards
Above the gilt table which holds the velvet-lined box
Containing the feet. He has left me alone
With souvenirs and my spondees.

Want ad in the *Mt. Rainier Gazette:* Come back, Scott,
Mother misses you. I will give you everything or nothing,
Whichever you need. Your bed is freshly made with striped sheets;
Spaghetti sauce and pies are in the freezer.
I love you. I have kept the feet in perfect condition.

the basic skills have been mastered
Our only enemy is uncertainty. In the act,
Even in the name to waver is to
    Trip. For instance: tightrope walker, a trifle awkward,
        But not until I thought of it did I discover
            R falling over W; and now my tongue
        Is always twisted by the word. You see
        You cannot say it once you
        Think about the process. And once you've thought you
                                                    cannot
    Say you will not think and stop your thoughts.
                The act of will defeats itself. And so, I fell
            In my final trial run . . . or walk.
                        Perhaps the feat—no, not the feet—
                Failed or was defeated by my hesitation.
But I am getting tangled up again.

    What I had planned to do was this:
    To play the last movement of Beethoven's Pathétique Sonata
                On the mid-point above Niagara Gorge.
            You see there is a grand tradition of tight-
Rope walking across the gorge,
                But this performance would have been something
            Quite unique. A tightrope man who is besides a skilled
                                                        pianist;
            Well, that is something new. And then simply to get
    The piano from the platform to the center demands a degree
        Of strength and balance beyond the norm. I had done it
Two weeks before at Quechee Gorge, but what had happened
Then should have given me pause: my memory lapsed
                About half-way through the movement and lapsed again
            Each time I started over, until I simply had to stick
    A dominant-tonic on and stop as if it were the end,

Which it was not, of course, but which it should have been.
          So two weeks later I paused and fell. I will not
       Go into the quarrels with my wife which came
    Before the fall. Or tell in detail
          How they weakened my confidence.
    It is enough to say I fell.

                    They had to amputate
                    But it was neat,
                    Just below both knees;
                    So I am now four feet
                    Instead of six feet tall,
                    Like Ferrer as Lautrec,
                    Except I really walk
                    On booted knees. You
                    Marvel at my attitude?
                    Well, I have had four
              Years in which to become detached.

And so the preamble concludes; the postamble
Begins. After a year in the hospital to heal
Internal injuries and train with my prosthetic feet,
I came home. My wife had found a job and with
My workman's compensation we could manage;
So it was not for money alone that I agreed
To teach the bearded lady. It was compassion,
A quality which comes with pain, or came for me.
She was losing the hair on her chin and as she'd had
Some tightrope training as a child wanted
    To take it up as an alternative profession.

  It was hard to build up her skill as fast as her hair fell out,
  But she was diligent and I compulsive
And by the time a small curled fall

79

Attached with spirit gum could no longer conceal
Her sparseness of beard, she was nearly ready,
    Totally ready in terms of what your average tightrope
                                                    walker

  Can do, but she was my pupil and average
      Was not enough. She couldn't play piano
        So that was out. I tell you that we agonized
          A lot to find that special thing. And then we never really
            Found it. It happened. I got divorced
And married her and she got pregnant. We both
          Knew right away a pregnant tightrope walker
            Was unique. I wish you could have seen her balance
                In the later months with that huge bulge in front;
  The crowds were absolutely quiet during the act
But when she finished her headstand
  And Rock-a-bye-baby ended with a fanfare
    The noise was louder than Niagara Falls.

      That this act had a built-in date for finishing
    Is evident. But we were ready, though not ready
  For the answer to a tightrope walker's prayers:
        Twins, the pairing for two arms, two breasts, two
                                                    buttocks,
      Two legs upon a single wire. Every night she walks,
        Balancing babies, they and she the product
  Of, respectively, my semen and my skill. I call myself
Thrice blessed and only sometimes worry
That she may hesitate. So far she never
Has. She never

                    Has.